Fatigue

How to be Free of Fatigue, Chronic Fatigue or Adrenal Fatigue and Cure it Forever without Resorting to Harmful Meds

Robert S. Lee

Contents

Chapter 1. A Look at Fatigue

Fatigue is an issue that many people face, and it's not an issue that you just have to deal with. Instead, you'll find that there are natural and herbal alternatives to help you fight fatigue. You'll find that it's actually a syndrome that can cause you to be tired all of the time. Just remember that chronic fatigue, adrenal fatigue and chronic fatigue syndrome are all different things, but herbal remedies can help at least a little with all three. You'll find that you can stop normal fatigue, even if you suffer from it often, in its tracks if you use natural and herbal solutions to keep you going.

Physical fatigue is where your muscles can't do things as easily as they used to, and this can include carrying bags or going up the stairs. It can cause weakness, even muscle weakness, and it makes you have a lack of strength. When doctors diagnose fatigue, they usually have to try a strength test to see if you're losing your ability to use your muscles like you use to. What you should know about fatigue, even chronic fatigue, is that it is common. Many people suffer from this persistent tiredness and weakness, and it can affect anyone from any walk of life.

However, you also need to know that there is a difference between sleepiness and fatigue, which many people will often confuse. Fatigue is a chronic condition, and sleepiness will come and go. Sleepiness is from a lack of stimulation, or because of a lack of sleep or at least quality sleep. It'll often be a symptom of a medical condition, but fatigue is different. It doesn't matter if you've had good sleep or not.

What it Affects:

Fatigue can affect your life, and it keep you from accomplishing what you want to do in the day or even over the week. When you don't have the energy to get out of bed, take a shower, or do the things you love, then you know you have an issue that you need to fix. Of course, you can fix it with herbal remedies. You'll find that fatigue is exhausting, makes you too tired, and it can cause listlessness.

Of course, there are symptoms of fatigues that you should look for as well. Bloating, tiredness, apathy, aching or sore muscles, irritability, indecisiveness, and loss of appetite are all related to chronic fatigue. You'll also notice poor immune system function, short term memory impairment, drowsiness, headaches, hallucinations, and even bad hand to eye coordination. It can even cause hallucinations, difficulty concentrating, apathy, and impaired hand-to-eye coordination.

Don't Deal with It:

You don't have to deal with fatigue. You can find a way to naturally fix it through habits and herbal remedies. You can also talk to your doctor to see what they suggest in treating your fatigue. Your doctor can diagnose chronic fatigue, and it'll help you to understand what you're dealing with so that you learn how to properly handle the issue.

Chapter 2. Natural Habits to Stack That Will Help

There are many habits that you can employ if you want to help fight your chronic fatigue quickly and effectively, and it'll help to make sure you're feeling better in no time. Some of these habits do take time to help you with improving your fatigue, but it will help to make sure that you'll stay away from a relapse or have your fatigue worsened.

Habit #1 Switch Coffee for Tea

You don't need coffee. It may be tempting if you're feeling tired and fatigued, but you'll find that it'll actually make it worse. Tea is a great choice to help warm you up and start feeling better quicker. You need to avoid some stimulants when it comes to fighting adrenal gland fatigue, which is one of the causes of chronic fatigue. So try to replace it with something else. Of course, you can always try a decaffeinated coffee as well. Just keep in mind that black tea has almost as much caffeine as coffee, so you should keep it out of the equation.

Habit #2 Eat Regularly

Food is a great way to help make sure that you're ready to face the day. You may want to include energizing snacks throughout the day, and you won't want to make your meals heavy, but they should be powerful. You'll find that your adrenal function, energy levels, and blood sugar are actually rather closely related. You should eat a breakfast that has a lot of fat and protein, and try to avoid stimulants and sugar if you want your adrenal function to go back to normal. It will help you to sleep better as well.

Habit #3 Meditate

It may seem simple, but you should meditate when you feel too stressed. Stress will only worsen any chronic fatigue, so it's important that you try and keep your stress levels under control if you don't want fatigue to take its toll. It'll help you to heal your adrenal glands by reducing your stress, and you can do it for fifteen minutes a day to start to feel better quickly. Of course, you can meditate for as long as you want, and you can do it before bed or when you get up in the morning. It doesn't even have to be a guided meditation. It can be as simple as breathing meditation.

Habit #4 Sleep on a Schedule

Sleeping on a schedule is going to help make sure that you're not as fatigued when you get up. When you're suffering from chronic fatigue, then you'll find that getting enough sleep is extremely important. If you aren't getting quality and quantity, then you won't be able to get up the next day very well, as it'll worsen your fatigue. Making sure that you have a bedtime routine really will help. You should have something to help you relax before you try to drift off to sleep, so that the quality won't be lacking.

Habit #5 Eat Meals on a Schedule

It's important that you keep on a schedule if you want to make sure that you aren't feeling down from your chronic fatigue. If you skip a meal, then your body is running on less energy than usual, and that's counterproductive when you're trying to fight fatigue. Make sure that you have meals on a schedule so that your body knows when to expect energy and that you get the energy you need to keep going.

Habit #6 Make Meals Small

It's also important that you make your meals small when you're fighting against chronic fatigue. When you eat larger meals, you're more likely to become lethargic and feel more fatigued than usual. It's better to eat six miniature meals daily than three large ones. It'll help to keep your energy levels up without too many drops and raises in your blood sugar levels.

Habit #7 Tea Before Bed

White tea or herbal tea is great before bed, and there are actually teas that you can use before bed that will help you sleep. You need to find a habit that will help you to get to sleep, and often a tea can do that. You don't need to have anything else, but water if you do. Never have caffeine or another stimulant before bed if you want to get both quality and quantity sleep. You also should take this time to power down. When you get your tea, you're going to want to turn off electronics and just sit there and enjoy it. Give yourself time to do nothing, and this will help you to wind down enough that your sleep isn't compromised. Remember to skip a glass of wine or a nightcap. Any alcohol will keep you from getting quality sleep, which is bad for those who suffer from chronic fatigue.

Habit #8 Skip the Smoke

Smoking will actually cause more fatigue as well, and if you are a sufferer from chronic fatigue, you need to cut the smoke out of your life. It'll irritate you and make you lethargic, which isn't going to help you to feel energized or happy. Not to mention that it's bad for your overall health, and it'll negatively impact your condition over time, worsening it. It can even cause your hormones to fluctuate which is bad for chronic fatigue. It even adds onto your stress levels and can make you lose sleep. So cut the smoke and replace it with a healthy hobby that will make quitting that much easier. For those who smoke, quitting is easier said than done, but it can be done. You can even talk to your doctor about getting various aids to help you quit the habit.

Habit #9 Listen to Music

Since stress and anxiety can actually cause your chronic fatigue to worsen, you'll find that listening to music can help. It'll help to make sure that you're relaxed, and you can even do so before bed or to start the day on the right foot. Twenty minutes of music that helps to calm you down and soothe you will help every day with fatigue. Without stress in your life, then your energy levels will already be up and won't be drained as much throughout the day. You can always listen to it more if you find that it helps as well.

Remember:

Habits are only meant to help you fight chronic fatigue. It won't actually cure it, but it will help to make sure that you're on the right track. When you add in herbal treatments and supplements, then it'll be a little easier to get through the day. Stack these habits so that you can fight fatigue on a regular basis.

Chapter 3. Teas to Pick You Up Quickly

Teas can be made for just about any problem, and chronic fatigue is able to be used. Teas are easy to make, and you can drink them hot or cold if you want to use them to help treat your chronic fatigue. It'll provide a pick me up, and it'll help to get you through the day.

Tea #1 Stinging Nettle

Stinging nettle tea can treat a variety of ailments, but it is also able to help treat chronic fatigue. It can also help with chest congestion, acne, and digestive issues. The best part is that stinging nettle tea is easy to make, and it's quick to work. You may notice results within ten to fifteen minutes.

Ingredients:

1. 1 Cup Water
2. 2 Teaspoons Stinging Nettle, Dried
3. 1 Teaspoon Honey, Raw

Directions:

1. Boil the water, and then turn off the heat. Place in the stinging nettle, and let it steep for fifteen to twenty minutes. Add in honey and drink warm or chilled depending on preference.

Tea #2 Cinnamon

Cinnamon is known to bring energy even when you're feeling drained, and it can help with blood sugar control and weight loss as well. It kicks in your metabolism and gives you the energy you need to get through the day. It's easy to make, so this honey and cinnamon recipe is flavorful and healthy.

Ingredients:

2. 2 Tablespoons Cinnamon, Ground
3. 1 ½ Teaspoons Honey, Raw
4. 1 Cup Water

Directions:

1. Boil the water, and then take it off heat. Add in the cinnamon, and let steep for ten to fifteen minutes.
2. Strain, and add in honey. You can drink warm or chilled. Many people like a splash of cream in this wonderful cinnamon tea, but it's up to preference.

Tea #3 Licorice Root

This is a licorice root tea, so if you like black licorice this is a great pick me up tea for you. It's simple to make, but it uses a dash of cinnamon to help give you that extra kick. Of course, many people skip it if you don't like the two flavors mixing. However, this blended tea will help you to fight fatigue quickly throughout the day.

Ingredients:

1. 1 ½ Teaspoons Licorice, Dried
2. ½ Teaspoon Cinnamon, Ground
3. 1 Teaspoon Honey, Raw

4. 1 Cup Water

Directions:

1. Boil the water, and then take off heat.
    Put in the licorice and cinnamon. Let it
    steep for eight to ten minutes.
2. Strain, and add honey. You can drink
    warm or chilled.

Tea #4 Lemon Balm

Lemon balm tea is also known to help pick you
up and help you to get though the day even
when you're suffering from chronic fatigue. It

helps your adrenal gland, and it is even known to help improve sleep. If you're using lemon balm tea to fight fatigue, you are going to want to use it three times daily.

Ingredients:

1. 2 Teaspoons Lemon Balm, Dried
2. 1 Teaspoon Honey, Raw
3. 1 Cup Water

Directions:

1. Boil the water, and then take it off heat. Add in the dried lemon balm and let steep for ten to twelve minutes.
2. Strain out the herbs and add in the honey to drink.

Tea #5 Ginger

Ginger tea is also a great way to help with chronic fatigue, and it can help your digestive system as well. It can help with nausea, and it can even help with motion sickness. If you have an upset stomach or need a boost, try some fresh ginger tea. It's even easy to get fresh ginger, so you don't have to deal with dried.

Ingredients:

1. 2 Tablespoons Ginger, Grated
2. ½ Teaspoon Lemon Juice, Fresh
3. 1 Teaspoon Honey, Raw
4. 1 Cup Water

Directions:

1. Boil the water, and then take it off heat. Put in the ginger and let it steep for eight to ten minutes.
2. Strain, and then add the lemon juice and honey. Stir and drink warm.

Tea #6 The Right Blend

You already know that lemon balm, ginger, and cinnamon will help you to fight chronic fatigue, but they make an interesting and tasty combination. You can drink this cup whenever you're feeling down, and it'll help you to stabilize your mood and it'll help to make sure that you can get through the day.

Ingredients:

1. 1 Teaspoon Ginger, Grated
2. 1 Teaspoon Honey, Raw
3. 1 Teaspoon Cinnamon, Ground
4. 1 ½ Teaspoons Lemon Balm, Dried

5. 1 Cup Water

Directions:

1. Boil your water before taking it off heat
    to add your lemon balm, cinnamon, and
    ginger. Let steep for twelve to fifteen
    minutes before straining.
2. You can drink warm or chilled, but add
    in honey before chilling if so.

Tea #7 Peppermint

Peppermint is a soothing and refreshing tea. It
helps with chronic fatigue, digestion,

heartburn, fever, and even cough. Peppermint tea is versatile and easy to get ahold of. Remember that if you don't have dried peppermint, you can use peppermint extract. Another added benefit from peppermint is that it helps to improve mental focus as well, which is usually disrupted when you're dealing with chronic fatigue.

Ingredients:

1. 2 Teaspoons Peppermint Leaves, Dried
2. 1 Teaspoon Honey, Raw
3. 1 Cup Water

Directions:

1. Boil your cup of water before putting in the peppermint leaves, allowing it too steep for six to eight minutes before straining.
2. Add in your honey and drink warm or chill and serve over ice. You can use fresh peppermint leaves to garnish.

Tea #8 Astragalus

Astragalus is a traditional Chinese herb that has a lot of benefits, and one of them is its ability to fight fatigue, including chronic fatigue. It's also a tea that you'd want to drink at least once daily if not twice daily. It's still easy to make, but you may have a hard time getting the herb. You can usually get it from a health and food store, but many people buy it online. It even helps to boost your immune system, which chronic fatigue can destroy.

Ingredients:

1. 3 Tablespoons Astragalus, Dried

2. ½ Teaspoon Cinnamon, Ground

3. 1 Teaspoon Honey, Raw

4. 1 Cup Water

Directions:

1. Boil your water before putting in astragalus and cinnamon, letting steep for ten to twelve minutes before straining.

2. Add in your honey and drink warm.

Tea #9 Green Tea & Ginseng

Green tea and ginseng are known to help fatigue and give you energy. It's great with honey, and you can add a fruit flavor, such as orange zest, if desired. You'll find that it helps to make it in advance, as this is a tea that tastes good when chilled, but it's up to you. It's best to drink it two to three times daily.

Ingredients:

1. 1 Cup Water
2. 2 Teaspoons Honey, Raw
3. 1 Teaspoon Ginseng, Powdered
4. 2 Tablespoons Green Tea Leaves

Directions:

1. Boil the water, and then put in the ginseng and green tea leaves. Let it steep for ten to twelve minutes after taking it off heat.

2. Strain, and then you can add in the honey before drinking hot or chill to drink later.

Tea #10 Lemon & Green Tea

Green tea is great for trying to get rid of your fatigue, and it will help you to clear your mind and set out for the day. Of course, lemon is known to help with stress and your digestive system, which will help you with chronic fatigue as well.

Ingredients:

1. 2 Tablespoons Green Tea Leaves
2. 1 Tablespoon Lemon Juice, Fresh
3. ½ Teaspoon Lemon Zest
4. 2 Teaspoons Honey, Raw
5. 1 Cup Water

Directions:

1. Boil your water, and then add in your lemon juice, lemon zest, and green tea when you remove it from heat. Let steep for six to eight minutes before straining.

2. Add honey and drink while warm, or
    chill it and serve it over ice.

Tea #11 The Fatigue Lifter

If you're looking for a way to fight your fatigue
quickly, you'll want to have this wonderful
blend that is a great pick me up in the morning.
It'll give you the energy you need to get through
the day while tasting great. It's good when
served hot or cold. Add more honey to sweeten
if desired.

Ingredients:

1. 1 Teaspoon Peppermint Leaves, Dried

2. ½ Teaspoon Ginseng Powder, Dried

3. ½ Teaspoon Lemon Juice, Fresh

4. 1 Teaspoon Maca Root, Ground & Dried

5. 1 Teaspoon Honey, Raw

6. 1 Cup Water

Directions:

1. Boil your cup of water, and then put in
    the peppermint, ginseng, lemon juice,
    and maca root. Take it off heat, and then
    you can let it steep for eight to ten
    minutes before straining.
2. Add honey and drink warm, or let chill
    and serve over ice.

Chapter 4. Foods to Work into Your Diet to Help

There are many different foods that you can add into your diet if you want to help with chronic fatigue as well. Here you'll find foods that are easy to add into your diet, and you'll even find a recipe for each which will help you with your chronic fatigue without sacrificing flavor.

Food #1 Cacao

Cacao powder is recommended with chronic fatigue because it helps to give you an energy boost while still nourishing both your brain and your heart. It's good for your overall health, including your digestive health. It's known to help get you through the day, and it can be added into smoothies or even baking. However, adding it to your breakfast smoothie or a snack is usually known to work best.

Example Recipe: *Cacao & Banana Blend*

Ingredients:

1. 1 Tablespoon Cacao Powder
2. 2 Teaspoons Honey, Raw

3. 2 Small Bananas, Sliced & Frozen

4. 1 Cup Strawberries, Fresh

5. ½ Cup Ice

6. ½ Cup Almond Milk, Vanilla & Sweetened

Directions:

1. Just put everything into the blender, and blend until smooth. Add more ice if needed to thicken. You can also add more honey if you want to sweeten the smoothie.

2.

Food #2 Kale

Kale, like most dark greens, is great when you're suffering from chronic fatigue. They contain vitamins, mineral, and antioxidants that are going to help you keep your body running even if you're tired, sleepy, or fatigued on a regular basis. It can even help to protect you from anemia, and they're even loaded down with iron to help your body.

Example Recipe: *Kale & Shrimp Dish*

This even has sweet potatoes in it, and it'll help to get enough kale into your diet. However, you'll also find that it can be added to a smoothie. This is a sweet and savory dish that you can use on a daily basis, and it's great for lunch or dinner. It even heat up well.

Ingredients:

1. 2 Tablespoons Olive Oil, Extra Virgin
2. ½ Teaspoon Red Pepper Flakes
3. ½ Cup Onion, Diced Small
4. 2 Cups Sweet Potatoes, Diced
5. 2 Cups Shrimp, Fresh
6. 3 Cups Kale, Chopped
7. ¼ Teaspoon Black Pepper, Ground
8. ½ Teaspoon Sea Salt, Fine
9. 3 Cloves Garlic, Minced

Directions:

1. Get out a medium saucepan, putting it over medium heat as you put in your extra virgin olive oil. Then add in your red pepper flakes and diced onion, cooking until the onions are golden and soft.
2. Add in your garlic, cooking for another thirty seconds.
3. Add in your sweet potatoes, cooking for about ten to fifteen minutes or until soft. You may need to add some water to steam.
4. Then, you can add in your shrimp, cooking until they turn pink, which usually takes two to four minutes.
5. Turn the heat to low, adding in your kale and stirring until wilted. Add in your salt and pepper, and serve.

Food #3 Blueberries

Blueberries are also wonderful to add into your diet if you're suffering from chronic fatigue. This is because chronic fatigue syndrome can lead to oxidative stress, which is bad for your body and your beauty. Blueberries helps to repair this damage, so you should always add it in whenever possible. Blueberries are extremely antioxidant rich.

Example Recipe: *Banana & Blueberry Bread*

You can eat this bread throughout the day, and it has a lot of antioxidants. You'll find that the blueberries are sweet, even if you use frozen one. When cooked into this bread, it's easy to have enough to help with oxidative stress, and it can be eaten throughout the day.

Ingredients:

1. 2 Cups Flour, All Purpose
2. ½ Teaspoon Sea Salt, Fine
3. 1 Cup White Sugar
4. ½ Cup Butter, Softened
5. 1 Teaspoon Baking Soda
6. 2 Large Eggs
7. 2 ½ Teaspoons Vanilla Extract
8. 2 Medium Ripe Banana, Mashed
9. 1 Cup Blueberries, Fresh

1. Start by heating your oven to 350, and then take three small loaf pans, greasing them to prepare them.
2. Take a medium bowl, mixing together the flour, salt, and baking soda.
3. In another large bowl, add butter and sugar, beating it together until it because light and fluffy. Add in an egg, and continue to blend, adding in vanilla extract. You'll then want to mix and beat in the banana before adding the flour mixture.
4. Keep beating until they combine to make a thick batter, and then tart to fold in your blueberries.
5. Pour into the loaf pans, and place in the oven. Let cook for thirty to thirty-five

minutes. They should be golden brown on the top.

Food #4 Lentils

Lentils are great plant based protein, and it's rich in minerals, helping to counteract the effects of fatigue. It'll help to give you the energy boost your need, and it's great to add into soups and even curries. When facing fatigue, you should always look for something that can boost your energy, and you can take soups with you in a thermos, so it makes a great lunch or even a dinner.

Example Recipe: *Spinach & Lentil Soup*

This is an easy spinach and lentil soup, and both spinach, as a dark green, and the lentils are going to help you with your fatigue. When you add in ginger, you have a powerful fatigue fighting recipe that's sure to help.

Ingredients:

1. 3 Cups Water
2. 5 Ounces Spinach
3. 1 ½ Teaspoons Cumin< Powder
4. ½ Teaspoon Ginger, Grated
5. 1 Teaspoon Smoked Paprika
6. ¼ Teaspoon Sea Salt, Fine
7. 15 Ounces Diced Tomatoes
8. 2 Cups Lentils, Dry

9. 5 Cloves Garlic, Minced

10. 3 Medium Carrots, Peeled & Chopped

11. 1 Medium Onion, Diced

Directions:

1. Dice your onion and carrot first, and then put it in a stockpot. It should be over medium heat, and you will need to sauté it for seven to eight minutes. Add in your ginger, cumin, paprika, salt, and garlic. Allow to sauté for one minute, and then add in your broth, water, tomatoes, and lentils. Increase the heat and let boil.

2. Once it boils, reduce the heat, and cover. It should simmer for twenty-five to thirty minutes. The lentils should be

tender. Make sure your spinach is chopped.

3. Right before you're done cooking, add in salt and spinach. Allow to wilt, and then serve.

Food #5 Coconut Oil

You'll find that many oils help with natural fatigue, and coconut oil is one of them. Another is olive oil or sesame oil. However, you can just cook with them, but you can sneak them into recipes as well. This is because fats are actually a great source of energy for your body. It can even help with blood pressure and your immune system health. Yu can even use flaxseed oil. This will even reduce the joint and muscle pain that can result from chronic

fatigue, so it helps with fatigue and its
symptoms.

Example Recipe: *Blended Smoothie*

This is a refreshing blend where you can sneak
coconut oil into it easily. You can use other oils
as well, but coconut oil blends best, and it has a
taste that you'll love with this smoothie. You
even use coconut milk, which is also known to
help with your muscles.

Ingredients:

1. 1 Cup Coconut Milk

2. 2 Teaspoons Honey, Raw

3. ¼ Cup Ice

4. 1 Cup Strawberries, Fresh

5. ½ Cup Mango Chunks, Frozen

6. 3 Tablespoons Coconut Oil

Directions:

1. Blend everything together until smooth
    and thick. Add more or less ice as
    needed.

Food #6 Salmon

Salmon, or any other animal protein, is a great way to go if you're looking to fight fatigue. Your body needs protein to get energy, and when you're fatigued that is the first thing you need. You need energy to get through the day.
Salmon can provide it, and it's a great source of omega-3 fatty acids as well.

Example Recipe: *Lemon & Herb Salmon*

This is a lemon and herb salmon that is easy to make, and you can pair it with any sides you want. You can use it as a part of dinner or on its own for lunch. Salmon is a healthy fish to eat whenever you want.

Ingredients:

1. 3 Ounces Butter
2. 1 Teaspoon Fresh Dill, Chopped
3. 4 Salmon Fillets, 5 Ounces Each
4. ¼ Teaspoon White Pepper, Ground
5. 2 Cloves Garlic, Chopped
6. 1 Tablespoon Parsley, Fresh & Chopped
7. 2 Teaspoons Lemon zest
8. 1 Teaspoon Sea Salt, Coarse

Directions:

1. All ingredients except the salmon can be placed in a small bowl and put into the microwave to melt. It should take thirty

to forty-five seconds. Stir so that they combine well.

2. Take your salmon fillet and lay them on a baking sheet that has been lined with parchment paper.

3. Take a pastry brush, and coat the salmon with your butter mixture. It should be spread evenly over the top.

4. Your oven will need set to 400 degrees. Cook it for ten to twelve minutes. The salmon should be cooked through, and it should flake easily.

Remember:

Remember to avoid any foods that may leave you tired, like foods with too many artificial ingredients or too much sugars. You'll want to choose foods that give you natural energy when you're trying to fight chronic fatigue syndrome. Including whole grains will also help you to fight chronic fatigue. Try to eat these foods on a daily basis throughout the day, and you'll find that it helps to prepare your body to fight fatigue, helping you to get through the day.

Chapter 5. Supplements That Really Do Work

There are supplements out there that can help you to fight chronic fatigue naturally as well, and many work as a quick and effective energy booster. You'll find that with these supplement you'll be feeling better in no time. Of course, when taking any pill, including supplements, you should make your doctor aware of what you're taking. Even natural supplements can interact with certain medication, prescription or over the counter. So make sure that your doctor knows about any change in your daily routine.

Supplement #1 Glycine

This is a supplement that is an amino, so it often will improve cognitive performance in one to two doses. It's found in a lot of foods, you'll get an extra boost when you get it in the supplement form. It can even help send the body to sleep, so if your fatigue is interrupting your quality of sleep, this is the supplement to help. Usually a recommended dosage is three grams, and better yet it's not considered an expensive supplement.

Supplement #2 Theanine

This is also able to be found in green tea, and it's another amino acid. It's great at helping with sleep, but don't mistake it for a sedative. It actually just improves the quality of sleep, helping you to feel more rested by the time that you wake up in the morning. The optimal dosage if you want to improve your sleep is 150 to 200 milligrams, and it should be taken a half hour to an hour before bed. It'll help you to feel rested enough to battle your chronic fatigue in the morning. It is also considered a relatively cheap supplement that is easy to add into your routine.

Supplement #3 Rhodiola Rosea

This is an adoptigen, as it's something that can help to desensitize you to a stressful event before it happens. It's great at treating metabolic burnout, and it's great at helping with cognition and even mild depression. It helps you to maintain proper levels of serotonin in your brain, which helps with your moods and hormones. If you're using it daily, you usually want to use 150 milligrams. However, you'll need to make sure that they're one percent salidrosidie while being three percent rosavins.

Supplement #4 Creatine

This is a dietary supplement that will actually help to promote effective energy juice, which also counteracts fatigue, especially from over exertion. It's known to help increase muscle size, and it will help make sure that your body will reserve glucose for later use, which will stave off the effects of fatigue. Many doctors agree that it's okay for long term use, but you should always ask your doctor if they think it's safe for you to use long term, as there is some controversy.

Supplement #5 Glucose

If you're looking for a stimulant then you might want to try glucose. It will help to improve performance, but it's also known to help your body maintain energy levels. You can add the glucose to water, and usually you add twenty to forty grams to sip during a workout, but your doctor can advise you on how to take it for your fatigue depending on the type of chronic fatigue that you're suffering from. You can add it safely to your diet.

Supplement #6 Melatonin

If you're having a hard time sleeping because of fatigue, you may actually not be getting the quality of sleep you need or the quantity. Melatonin is known to help with both quality and quantity when it comes to sleep, helping to make sure that you're rested so that you can start your day off on the right foot. This will help with your fatigue over time. When there's too much light in your bedroom your body may not want to sleep or it may not be able to, but melatonin can help.

Supplement #7 Vitamin C

Vitamin C is actually extremely important if you're suffering from fatigue. If you lack vitamin C, then you can suffer from fatigue even more. It can help to prevent fatigue that is caused by various infection, which does include chronic fatigue for many people. Vitamin C can also increase the way your body absorbs iron from the digestion track, which can help with fatigue and anemia, which can cause fatigue. Without vitamin C you are much more likely to have allergies as well, which can worsen fatigue, and you will have more stress because you won't have a sufficient adrenal gland function.

Supplement #8 Vitamin E

Vitamin E is also great if you're suffering from fatigue, and this is because it helps with the immune system response, which can keep fatigue at bay. It is also an important antioxidant which will help to protect your cells, and it can even prevent anemia. It can also help people who suffer from vitamin E. Vitamin E is great to put into your diet, and it's relatively safe with various over the counter and prescription medications.

Supplement #9 Zinc

Zinc is actually really important when it comes to helping to combat fatigue, and it can help you to improve your muscle strength as well as muscle endurance. It can help to enhance immune function, which will help reduce fatigue. It can also help with metabolism and digestion. You can use food to get zinc, but it is often hard to get enough in your diet. It comes from whole grain wheat bran, pumpkin seeds, wheat germ, and even high protein foods, but if you are deficient in zinc foods that are high in it may not be enough.

Supplement #10 Potassium

Potassium deficiencies are common, and you'll find that potassium helps to increase energy and vitality. It helps with muscular weakness as well as fatigue, and it can help you even if you're battling with chronic fatigue. It can help restore energy levels, and it can keep your muscles from hurting, which is what many people experience when battling with chronic fatigue. It even helps with maintaining a nervous system function as well as a healthy heart rate.

Supplement #11 Calcium

Chronic fatigue can cause stress, and calcium can help with that as well as helping with the fatigue itself. Calcium can help with anxiety, nervous tension, and even emotional upset. If you don't have the amount of calcium you need it can cause mood swings, fatigue, and muscular irritability as well as cramps. Calcium is essential to your diet, and it can be added into your regime with little to no repercussion. Of course, like any supplement, you should still ask your doctor before adding it into your daily routine.

Supplement #12 Maca Root

If you're dealing with chronic fatigue, you may want to try maca root. Maca root helps with cortisol regulation, which helps with stress and anxiety. It can also help with blood sugar levels. It can help for adrenal fatigue and it helps your body to make use of its low hormone levels, which will fight fatigue effectively.

Supplement #13 Licorice Root

Licorice root can actually be taken in supplement form, and it supports adrenal gland fatigue, helping with chronic fatigue. You can, of course, use licorice root tea, but it won't always help as effectively as the supplement, and you may not like the taste. That's where licorice root supplements come in, and you can always ask your doctor before adding it into your daily routine. It increases your endurance, and it helps to retain energy levels, which will help you to fight fatigue throughout the day. It is even known to stimulate hormone production which helps may people. However, you should be aware that licorice root can raise your blood pressure, especially when taken in a supplement, so your doctor must be aware, like with any supplement, before you add it into your routine.

Chapter 6. Essential Oil Blends to Help Out

Essential oil blends can be made in advance, and they work great if you're looking for something to help you combat your chronic fatigue quickly. When you get a roller container to carry them in, it's easy to use them anywhere you go. This will help to make sure that you have that pick me up whenever you need it to help you get through the day. Most people will find rollerball tubes at a local health and beauty store, but you can always order them online if necessary. It's like putting on a perfume or cologne directly to your skin, and you can roll it on anywhere you need it with these smell good oils and all of their benefits.

Essential Oil Blend #1 Exhaustion & Fatigue

You should use a ten millimeter rollerblade for most recipes, and this recipe is no different. It'll help you to fight exhaustion immediately, and it smells great doing it. Eucalyptus essential oil is great for muscle aches, and it can help to stimulate you which will help with clarity and mental awareness. You'll find that rosemary essential oil can also help with fatigue, and it can even help to aid in memory. Grapefruit essential oil is great for muscle fatigue as well as arthritis.

Ingredients:

1. 20 Drops Eucalyptus Essential Oil

2. 15 Drops Rosemary Essential Oil

3. 3-5 Drops Grapefruit Essential oil

4. Sweet Almond Oil

Directions:

1. Pour all of your essential oils into the bottle, and then finish topping off with the carrier oil. Shake well before using.

Essential Oil Blend #2 Fatigue & Aching Muscles

Peppermint essential oil is a great pick me up, and it helps with mental fatigue. You'll find that it helps to keep you awake as well, and when balanced with lavender, you'll find that it can help with fatigue as well by helping with the stress and anxiety that fatigue can bring. This blend smells great, and it'll put your mind at ease while keeping you awake. If you're worried about your coconut oil becoming too solid, you can always add a few drops of sweet almond oil as the carrier oil as well.

Ingredients:

1. 30 Drops Peppermint Essential Oil

2. 20 Drops Coconut Oil

3. 30 Drops Lavender Essential Oil

Directions:

1. Put everything into the roller bottle and then shake well to blend. Apply it directly to any area where you feel the effects of sore muscle or fatigue.

Essential Oil Blend #3 Fatigue Diffuser

You already know that rosemary and peppermint are great pick me ups, and they'll help to diffuse fatigue quickly. Peppermint is great for mental awareness, and it'll help with stress and mental fatigue quickly. Lemongrass essential oil also helps with stress and fatigue, including chronic fatigue.

Ingredients:

2. 15 Drops Rosemary Essential Oil
3. 15 Drops Peppermint Essential Oil
4. 8 Drops Lemongrass Essential Oil
5. Coconut Oil

Directions:

1. Mix everything together, putting it in the roller bottle and then top off with coconut oil. Shake well before using.

Essential Oil Blend #4 A Quick Pick Me Up

Cypress is known to help with emotional security as well as fatigue. It's even antiviral, and it'll help to make sure that you don't get sick from the fatigue suppressing your immune system. Basil is also great for fatigue, as it's a mental stimulant. It also helps with depression and anxiety. Of course, peppermint helps with mental clarity as well as to wake you up quickly.

Ingredients:

1. 15 Drops Cypress Essential Oil
2. 15 Drops Basil Essential Oil
3. 8 Drops Peppermint Essential Oil
4. Sweet Almond Oil

Directions:

1. Mix everything together, and then top
    off with almond oil in the rollerball
    bottle. Shake well before using.

Essential Oil Blend #5 Wake Me Up

When you're dealing with fatigue, especially
chronic fatigue, you'll find that sometimes you
just need to be able to wake up and wake up
quickly. This is what this essential oil blend
helps with, giving you the energy you need to
get through the day despite the fatigue that
you're feeling. You already know that basil and
peppermint will help to wake you up, and rose

essential oil is known to help relieve your stress which in turn can help you to relieve fatigue. Lemon is also known to help, just like lemongrass essential oil, as it helps with stress as well.

Ingredients:

1. 20 Drops Basil Essential Oil
2. 20 Drops Lemon Essential Oil
3. 10 Drops Peppermint Essential Oil
4. 5 Drops Rose Essential Oil
5. Sweet Almond Oil

Directions:

1. Mix all essential oils together in the rollerball bottle, and then top off with the sweet almond oil. Mix well before applying.

Essential Oil Blend #6 Sleep Quality Blend

Often, a contributing factor to fatigue, especially chronic fatigue, is lack of quality of sleep even if you are getting enough sleep. Rose and lavender help to relieve fatigue by helping relax your body and remove the tension. Marjoram essential oil is also a great way to help relax you before bed since it's a muscle relaxer as well. This blend is sure to help you get the quality of sleep that you need to help you battle chronic fatigue on a regular basis.

Ingredients:

1. 20 Drops Lavender Essential Oil
2. 10 Drops Rose Essential Oil
3. 5 Drops Marjoram Essential Oil
4. Coconut Oil

Directions:

1. Mix all essential oils together in the rollerball bottle, and then top with the coconut oil. Mix well.

Essential Oil Blend #7 Calm Down & Pick Me Up

Sometimes you just need to calm down before getting picked up. That's why there is roman chamomile and peppermint. Of course, grapefruit essential oil will help to combat your fatigue immediately, and peppermint will help with mental clarity along the way.

Ingredients:

1. 5-8 Drops Grapefruit Essential Oil
2. 20 Drops Peppermint Essential Oil
3. 10 Drops Roman Chamomile Essential Oil
4. Coconut Oil
5. Sweet Almond Oil

Directions:

1. Mix all essential oils together in the rollerball bottle before topping it off with coconut oil and sweet almond oil. Make sure to mix well.

Essential Oil Blend #8 Focus from Fatigue

This is a great essential oil blend to help you focus. You already know that peppermint will pick your mind up and keep you focused, but so will wild orange essential oil. One of the best parts is that it smells great doing it. It can even help with stress, depression, and anxiety. It works in a diffuser as well.

Ingredients:

1. 20 Drops Wild Orange Essential Oil
2. 20 Drops Peppermint Essential Oil
3. Sweet Almond Oil

Directions:

1. Just mix all of the essential oils together, and then put it in the rollerball bottle.
2. Top it off with the sweet almond oil, and then mix well before use. Shake it every time you use it.

Chapter 7. Extra Tips to Help Out

There are still many tips and tricks that you can employ to help you fight chronic fatigue and start feeling better quickly. These are changes to your daily routine that will help you, and sometimes it's just an outlook. Either way, by using these tips, it'll help to make sure that you'll get where you need to be to fight your fatigue and go through the day naturally and a little happier and healthier.

Tip #1 Try to Avoid Overexertion

If you don't want a relapse or to make your chronic fatigue worse, then you're going to need to try and avoid overexertion to the best of your ability. Even when you're feeling well, you shouldn't try to do too much or you'll relapse and start to feel bad again. You still have a medical condition that you need to be careful of so that you aren't trying to push past your energy levels and overextend yourself.

Tip #2 Keep Stress Away

The way you choose to do this is still up to you, but if you want to fight chronic fatigue and keep away from a relapse if you're feeling better, then you're going to need to keep it away. Stress will drain your energy, and it can worsen chronic fatigue if you have it, including the symptoms. Try various relaxation techniques until you find something that will help you to keep stress at bay.

Tip #3 Keep a Journal

You'll want to keep a journal so that you keep track of all of your triggers. There are things, including activities and perhaps people who are emotionally draining, that will affect your chronic fatigue and even worsen it. Often, it's hard to see what your triggers are, but when you write it down it'll help to make sure that you can avoid these triggers. Make sure you know what causes your stress, how much rest you're getting, and what daily activities may be making it worse.

Tip #4 Exercise Enough But Not Too Much

You can't avoid exercise completely, but you need to make sure that if you suffer with chronic fatigue that you aren't overexerting yourself. You need exercise to stay healthy, but it doesn't mean that you need to overextend yourself if you're having a hard time with fatigue in the first place. When most people might be able to handle an hour or thirty minutes, someone fighting with chronic fatigue may only be able to handle fifteen minutes of exercise at a time. If you're already keeping a journal, you'll be able to keep track of when you're having more trouble than other times when it comes to exercise being too much.

Tip #5 Keep Hydrated

You may not think that water makes that much of a difference, but it does. Water can make the difference between having energy and not having it. Dehydration will zap your energy, and you won't be able to do anything without even more fatigue. When you drink enough water, you're more likely to have more energy, and it'll increase alertness and concentration.

Tip #6 Maintain a Healthy Weight

There are many different ways to help fight fatigue, but you're more likely to feel the effects of chronic fatigue if you aren't at a healthy weight. Try to reach and stay at a healthy weight if you want to help keep the symptoms of your fatigue down. Of course, if you're eating a diet that helps with fatigue, it should help you to make sure that you're at a healthy weight as well.

Remember:

Fighting chronic fatigue can be hard, and it's an uphill battle where you don't always see an end. If you're dealing with chronic fatigue, then you need to try and make sure that you are always finding a way to help alleviate stress and anxiety to help you keep moving forward. There are many natural ways and herbal remedies that you can implement to make sure that your fatigue is manageable and under control. One of the most important parts of fighting chronic fatigue is not giving up so that you can find what's right for you to work into your schedule and how to handle it.